Diabetes

How to Manage, Prevent and Reverse!

Control Blood Sugar Through Superfoods!

Peggy Chan

ISBN: 978-1539716389

Disclaimer

The information contained in this book is not designed to replace or take the place of any form of medicine or professional medical advice. The information in this book has been provided for educational and entertainment purposes only. The information contained in this book has been compiled from sources deemed reliable and it is accurate to the best of the Author's knowledge; however, the Author cannot guarantee its accuracy and validity and cannot be held liable for any errors or omissions. Upon using the information contained in this book, you agree to hold harmless the author from and against any damages, costs, and expenses, including any legal fees, potentially resulting from the application of any of the information provided by this guide. The disclaimer applies to any damages or injury caused by the use and application, whether directly or indirectly, of any advice or information presented, whether for breach of contract, tort, neglect, personal injury, criminal intent, or under any other cause of action. You agree to accept all risks of using the information presented inside this book. You need to consult a professional medical practitioner or get medical advice before using any of the suggested remedies, techniques, or information in this book.

Dedication

This book is dedicated to my late parents, who were diabetics, and to my diabetic siblings. It is also dedicated to all diabetics.

A Gift for You

Thank you for reading my book. As a token of appreciation, I would like to give you a list of the Glycemic Index of food which you can download and print out. This will help you to make healthy choices when grocery shopping for your meals.

To get your gift, go to:

http://www.peggychan.online/gi-food-list-signup/

Contents

Introduction

During a routine check-up at the public hospital, the doctor cautioned me, saying, "Diabetes is one disease you never want to have, if you can prevent it."

"Why?" I asked, my heart in my mouth, as my parents had it and my two younger brothers also had it.

"It's a progressive disease and it leads to many life-threatening complications. I'm sending you for a blood test to check your sugar levels. Remember to fast the night before you do the test the following morning."

My blood test was scheduled in two weeks' time and the doctor would see me two weeks after that.

In the meantime, I did some research on Diabetes. One fact stood out.

More and more people are getting Diabetes. The people prone to Diabetes are usually middle-aged and most of them become diabetic in their mid-fifties. However, these days, people as young as thirty are suffering from Diabetes.

Can it be prevented?

If I were to be diagnosed as a diabetic, would I be doomed to develop the complications mentioned by the doctor? Between a confirmed diagnosis of the disease and the complications leading from it, is there anything that can be done to arrest its progression? Could I take any preventive measures to stop the disease from getting worse and negatively impacting my life?

When I saw the doctor again, he confirmed that I had Diabetes. When he saw my reaction, he reassured me, "Don't worry, it's not the end of the world. This is what I want you to do."

In this book, I share with you my findings on Diabetes, and my life as a diabetic. I was diagnosed more than ten years ago and I'm still enjoying a good quality of life. If you aren't already a diabetic or if you are a pre-diabetic, there is information in this book that will be of great benefit to you.

You will learn:

- what Diabetes is

- the different types of Diabetes

- the causes of Diabetes

- whether or not you have Diabetes

- the different life-threatening complications that develop as the disease progresses

- what you can do to prevent Diabetes or reverse it in the early stages

- how to manage Diabetes if you are already a diabetic

- what you can eat to maintain blood sugar control

- and many other things of benefit to your overall health

As you apply what you learn in this book, you will experience the rewards that I'm still enjoying today, a quality life that comes with better health and seeing my grandchildren growing up.

Now, isn't that something to look forward to?

Diabetes: What Is It?

Diabetes is a progressive metabolic disease brought about by the high levels of blood sugar in the body. Now you may ask, "What is blood sugar? How does it get high?"

Another name for blood sugar is glucose, and our bodies need this glucose, as it is the main source of energy for our cells. Our bodies make glucose from foods that contain carbohydrates, such as bread, rice, pasta, potatoes and fruit, etc.

The glucose is carried in the blood to our cells. However, it needs a hormone called insulin to enable the glucose to enter the cells. This hormone, insulin, is produced by the pancreas.

Insulin helps our blood to carry glucose to all of the cells in our bodies, to provide the energy that the cells need, in order to keep our bodies functioning.

Sometimes the pancreas doesn't make enough insulin, or the insulin doesn't work properly.

Then the glucose remains in our blood, leading to high blood glucose levels or high sugar levels, which can cause Prediabetes, or Diabetes and other health issues linked to Diabetes.

Now let's see how many types of Diabetes there are. I didn't know there were different types of Diabetes until I did some research on it.

Types of Diabetes

Before we go into the different types of Diabetes, you will be relieved to know that you don't suddenly develop Diabetes. You don't get it overnight. You would first find yourself diagnosed with Prediabetes.

What is Prediabetes?

How would you know whether you are suffering from Prediabetes?

Well, if you lead a sedentary life and hardly exercise, if you are overweight and have accumulated fat around your waist and abdomen, you could very likely be pre-diabetic. However, you wouldn't know unless you go for a blood test. That's why many people don't know that they are pre-diabetic and at very high risk for developing Diabetes. A blood test will confirm if this is the case.

Before anyone can have a blood test to check their sugar levels, they need to fast for at least 8 hours before the test.

A **normal blood sugar reading,** from a test done after fasting, is in the range of **3.8-5.8mmol/L or between 70–105 mg/dL**. So a person with this reading is not diabetic.

If blood sugar levels are higher than normal, but not so high as to be considered diabetic, that indicates pre-diabetes.

A reading of **6.1–7mmol/L or between 110–126mg/dL,** after fasting, **indicates impaired glucose tolerance** or, in other words, the person is **pre-diabetic**.

Moreover, if family members already have Diabetes, there is a higher risk of developing Prediabetes. A pre-diabetic can either reverse their condition or they can develop Diabetes, down the road.

If the **fasting blood sugar reading is more than 7 or 126mg/dL on 2 separate occasions**, they can be confirmed as a **diabetic**.

Is there any way you can avoid getting Prediabetes?

Yes, definitely, but let's leave that to a later chapter.

Let's consider the different types of Diabetes first.

There are three types of Diabetes:

- Type I Diabetes or Insulin Dependent Diabetes

- Type 2 or Diabetes Mellitus

- Gestational Diabetes

Type 1 Diabetes

This is an auto-immune disease. The body's own immune system produces antibodies, which destroy the insulin-producing cells in the pancreas. So the pancreas cannot produce any insulin.

However, the body needs insulin in order to function. Thus people who have Type 1 Diabetes must have insulin every day in order to live. They require daily insulin which is administered by way of injections or from an insulin pump which releases insulin at programed times through a needle embedded in the skin.

Unfortunately, nothing can be done to prevent Type 1 Diabetes and neither has a cure been found at this present time.

Type 2 Diabetes

Type 2 Diabetes is also known as **Diabetes Mellitus or Adult Onset Diabetes**. This is often called a life style disease and we will talk about why, in a later chapter.

Type 2 diabetes usually begins with insulin resistance, which is the body's inability to effectively use the insulin produced by the pancreas. Somehow, the glucose cannot enter the cells to be converted into energy for your body's needs. As a result, the glucose remains in the blood and the glucose levels rise. The high blood sugar levels cause the insulin producing beta cells in the pancreas to produce more insulin. Eventually these cells become impaired and can't make enough insulin to meet the body's demands. When the pancreas does not produce enough insulin for the body's needs, the sugar levels in the blood will rise.

The high blood sugar levels lead to Prediabetes which, if nothing is done to treat it, eventually develops into Diabetes.

Gestational Diabetes

Gestational diabetes can develop during pregnancy, usually during the second trimester, when the body does not produce enough insulin to meet the expectant mother's needs. However, once the baby is born, the mother's insulin requirement returns to normal and the Diabetes goes away.

Who is likely to suffer from Diabetes?

Type 1 Diabetes

It is mainly children who have Type 1 Diabetes, due to genetic factors. They are born with it. There are also adolescents who suffer a sudden onset of the disease, possibly brought about by a viral infection, which triggers the immune system to destroy the insulin-producing cells in the pancreas. These people will have to be on insulin for the rest of their natural lives. However, with good sugar level control, they can lead normal lives.

Type 2 Diabetes

If both parents are diabetic, their offspring have a very high chance of developing the disease in later life.

Diabetics are predominantly the middle-aged people and the elderly but, these days, younger people, and even children, are diagnosed with Diabetes because of their poor eating habits and over-consumption of the wrong types of food.

Gestational Diabetes

5 to 8 % of all pregnant women will develop Gestational Diabetes in the 24th to 28th week of pregnancy.

A woman who is pregnant needs three times the normal amount of insulin. When the pancreas does not produce enough insulin to meet her requirements, she will develop Gestational Diabetes.

Women in the family way who are over 30 years old and whose family members have diabetes are at risk too. Pregnant women who gain excessive weight, and are obese, will very likely develop Gestational Diabetes

How Do You Know If You Have Diabetes?

Well, if you have some of the following symptoms, you can be almost certain that you have either Pre-diabetes or Diabetes.

- Always thirsty

- Always feeling hungry and craving sweet things

- Feeling fatigued or lethargic

- Very drowsy throughout the day

- Frequent need to pass urine

- Blurred vision

- Cuts or injuries that take a long time to heal

- Tingling feelings or numbness in the hands and feet

- Itchy skin, with or without rashes

- Leg cramps

- Low libido

- Mood swings

- Headaches

- Dizziness

- Weight loss

If you have more than one of the above symptoms you need to consult a doctor to establish whether or not you have diabetes.

In an earlier chapter, you read that a person is pre-diabetic before he develops Diabetes. Unfortunately, a pre-diabetic often doesn't have any symptoms, so he doesn't realize that he has Prediabetes until it is too late. Then he is confirmed to be a diabetic.

This was what happened to me. I was obese, because I ate lots of sweet stuff, especially ice cream because, where I live, it's very, very hot all the year round, and I drank lots of ice-cold carbonated drinks. I didn't realize I was pre-diabetic as I had no way of knowing. I didn't know the symptoms of Diabetes. No one goes for a blood test unless there is reason to.

Even though my parents were diabetic, I didn't see the need to be careful about what I ate or drank. I ate whatever took my fancy and with seconds to boot! I loved food, especially the sweet stuff and I had that attitude; you know, the attitude that it's always other people that get it and that it wouldn't happen to me. Well, it finally happened to me! I was way beyond the pre-diabetic stage. I had Diabetes!!

So please, please, if you have any of the symptoms listed above, go to a doctor and ask to have your blood tested for Diabetes. If you're diagnosed as a pre-diabetic, the chances of you being able to reverse that condition and normalize your blood sugar levels are good.

How Does One Get Diabetes?

Remember, in an earlier chapter, I mentioned that Diabetes is said to be a lifestyle disease? What does this mean?

The following are indicative of the unhealthy lifestyles that people generally lead today which put them at risk for Prediabetes and Diabetes.

1. Smoking, as in heavy smoking and chain smoking.

2. Drinking, which goes beyond social drinking.

3. Obesity, and excessive intake of sugar in the form of carbonated drinks, sodas, confectionery, refined carbohydrates, etc.

4. Sedentary lifestyle, where exercise is not part and parcel of life.

5. Insufficient sleep—i.e. less than 5 hours' sleep a day, due to late nights

6. Stress, arising from worry, anxiety, tensions or grief, whether in the workplace or on the home front.

7. Overweight, with a BMI of 25 and above.

8. Having excess fat around the waist and abdomen, e.g. men whose waists measure more than 90 cm and women whose waists are more than 80 cm.

Are you familiar with any or all of the above? Are any of them a part of your lifestyle? Are you overweight or obese? Are you a couch potato?

Leading such an unhealthy lifestyle raises the risk of developing full-blown Diabetes.

What Does Diabetes Lead To?

Remember what the doctor said? That Diabetes can lead to life-threatening conditions? Let's see what these are.

Diabetics, both Type 1 and Type 2, who do not control their blood sugar levels, but continue to lead unhealthy lifestyles, are at risk for the following:

1. heart disease

2. stroke

3. nerve disease, which can lead to amputation of the feet and even the lower limbs

4. kidney failure

5. certain types of cancer, such as liver, pancreas, colorectal, breast, bladder

6. blindness

7. poor blood circulation

8. muscle pain

9. lean muscle loss

10. inflammatory arthritis

11. depression

12. premature death

All the above are life threatening and very frightening too!!

A **heart attack** will leave you weak (if it doesn't kill you!) and your lifestyle will be compromised. You will no longer be able to enjoy the kind of life you had before your heart attack.

Strokes are the result of having high blood pressure that is left untreated. Many people do not realize that they have high blood pressure until they are felled by a stroke. This is why it is also known as the silent killer. Diabetics have elevated blood pressure which puts them at risk for strokes.

A stroke will leave you incapacitated and dependent on care givers for the rest of your natural life, unless you suffer further strokes that hopefully will end your life and put you out of your misery. Otherwise, imagine being bedridden, unable to communicate because you are paralysed on one side of your body, unable to perform anything for yourself, suffering from bed sores, etc. for the rest of your natural life span.

Quite unthinkable and horrifying, isn't it?

Nerve damage, or peripheral neuropathy, is when you can't feel anything in your hands and legs. Poor blood circulation is a contributory factor. You feel numbness in your hands and legs. Prior to that stage, your skin would have been itchy and rashes would have appeared. You would have felt tingling sensations or little currents of electricity shooting down your calves and painful leg cramps, even toe cramps where one toe curled above another and like me, you would have had a difficult and painful time, trying to uncurl that stubborn, offending toe.

When you injure your toes or feet, while wearing open foot wear, the wounds can often lead to ulcers which don't heal because of Diabetes. This means you could end up having your toes, or your feet amputated because of the ensuing gangrene.

Can you imagine a life with stumps instead of your feet?

Kidney failure is the result of overworked kidneys. High blood sugar levels in the blood stress the kidneys. Over a period of time, this leads to kidney disease and then the kidneys fail. This will necessitate dialysis to cleanse the blood. A patient on dialysis is on the machine three times a week for a prolonged period of a few hours each time. This means you can't go for holidays because you need to be on the dialysis machine three times a week. It will come to a stage when dialysis doesn't work anymore and your only chance to live would be a kidney transplant. The scarcity of donors, a long waiting list in the hospital and the high costs of such transplant surgery are very discouraging.

Cancer is a disease that is not only catastrophic to the sufferer but also to immediate family members. It is very painful to contemplate as I lost my diabetic parents and two sisters to this disease. It is a terrible disease that many people succumb to, these days.

In Diabetes, **blindness** creeps up on you as a result of progressive macular degeneration of the optic nerve. Diabetics suffer blurred vision because of damage to blood vessels in the eye.

This can lead to loss of vision or diabetic retinopathy. Imagine not being able to see the beautiful sights around us! People who don't know that they're diabetic often think that blurred vision is part of growing old, hence they don't do anything about it. By the time they do get to a doctor, it's too late to save their sight.

Diabetics **lose lean muscle mass** and this aggravates the situation because there is less tissue to absorb the glucose. They are also more vulnerable to muscle injury, injury to ligaments and joint injury. Some diabetics may also suffer from **inflammatory arthritis**.

When a diabetic suffers from a few of the above conditions, it will be no surprise to find them in a state of **depression**. Their poor health, which is deteriorating by the day, pushes them into a state of mind where they feel terrified and at a loss. Their anxiety levels and worries escalate, as they wonder how to cope with their situation. **Stress** makes them sink deeper into depression, which, as we are aware, **can kill**.

A **premature death** at a time when many people are enjoying a life span of four score or more is painful to contemplate. A breadwinner being cut off in the prime of one's life is devastating to family members, especially if there are young children in the family. The consequences are far reaching.

Now it is clear why the doctor said that Diabetes is one disease no one should have. He should also have clarified that it is preventable if people are made aware of its terrible consequences and how to avoid getting the disease. But then, doctors are overworked and don't have the time to educate patients. Too many other patients are outside waiting for their turn to see the doctor.

Now that we know that Diabetes can lead to such terrible complications, is there anything that we can do to avoid them?

Can we prevent Diabetes?

Of course, there is much that you can do to prevent Diabetes if you are still in the clear!

Let's see how and what we can do about it, in the next chapter.

What Can You Do About It?

There are many things you can do to make sure that you won't suffer the complications described in the previous chapter.

If you are not diabetic, and you want to prevent Diabetes from becoming your life-long companion, you will want to adopt the same measures that a diabetic should take.

The first and most important step is to **change your present lifestyle.**

Take stock of your current situation.

What is your BMI? (Body Mass Index)

How do you calculate your BMI?

$$\frac{\text{Weight (kg)}}{\text{Height x Height (m)}} = \textbf{BMI}$$

So – get your weight in Kg, measure your height in metres, multiply your height by itself, and divide your weight by that number – the answer is your BMI.

World Health Organisation classification of BMI:

Underweight:	18.5 and below
Normal range:	18.5 – 24.99
Overweight:	Over 25
Obese:	Over 30

Apart from checking your BMI to find out whether you are overweight or obese, you can also check your waist measurements. Men, if your waist measures more than 40 inches, you are obese. Ladies, you are obese if your waist is more than 35 inches.

If you are overweight or obese, you need to lose weight, otherwise you risk developing Diabetes and heart disease, both of which will lead to a premature death.

How can you lose weight?

First of all, think about your lifestyle. Are you an active person?

Or do you find yourself sitting in front of the computer or telly, most of the time?

I don't want to frighten you, but leading such a sedentary lifestyle will lead to obesity (a fat belly and a big waistline), high blood cholesterols (high LDL and low HDL) and triglycerides, high blood pressure and high blood sugar. This cluster of health conditions is known as metabolic syndrome and it will eventually lead to Diabetes.

If you are physically inactive, you do have to find a way of getting rid of the excess weight you are carrying. Think of the years of life you could lose if you don't get rid of that weight. Think of how you will look in another few years with more flab and more fat on you!

Now, now, don't jump to the idea that you need to go on a crash diet to lose weight! I'm not advising you to do that because it won't work. Engaging in regular physical activity is the way to go.

This is especially so if you want to prevent Diabetes. Studies have ascertained that regular exercise improves sensitivity to insulin and increases lean muscle mass so that fat can be burned. This translates into weight loss.

You need to have a regular exercise routine. Before we go into the types of exercises that you can do, let's check out the benefits of exercise.

Once you see how beneficial exercise is, you'll definitely want to include it as part of your daily life.

So what are the benefits of regular exercise?

There are so many benefits.

First of all, it reduces the risk of heart disease. It lowers blood pressure and improves heart function. It also helps to lower blood cholesterol and triglyceride levels and it raises the good cholesterol or HDL.

It increases muscle strength and muscle mass, as well as giving you better flexibility. It also strengthens our bones by increasing bone density and prevents osteoporosis.

Exercise also helps us to destress and to relax, so that we can enjoy a better quality of sleep.

Our immune system is also strengthened, because more oxygen is delivered effectively throughout the body as a result of better blood circulation.

It can lift us out of depression, because exercise makes us feel good. Have you experienced a rush of good feeling after an enjoyable workout?

It also promotes weight loss. Long after an exercise session, our bodies continue to burn calories. Exercise also helps to suppress our appetite.

We feel more energetic and happy, because exercise helps our digestion and also aids in elimination of toxic wastes from our body. Constipation will be a thing of the past.

It improves sexual function.

Exercise promotes good health and diabetics definitely benefit from regular exercise, as it can also reduce blood sugar levels.

What kinds of exercise can you do?

Remember that the exercise should be regular and moderate. You don't want to over exert yourself and fall sick. Bear in mind that whatever you exercise you do, moderation is key.

The types of exercise we should include in our exercise regimen are:

A. Aerobic

B. Strength training

C. Stretching

A. What constitutes aerobic exercise?

Examples of aerobic exercise are:

- Walking briskly (4 to 5 days in a week)

- Cycling

- Swimming

- Low impact indoor exercise using exercise equipment, e.g. treadmill, stationary bicycling

- Dancing: line dancing, folk dancing,

- Jazzercise

- Golfing

- Gardening

- Tennis

Since many diabetics are in the middle age range or elderly, I suggest daily walks. Let's delve more into walking as a form of exercise.

The best time to walk is in the early morning when the air is fresh and it is still cool. Walk briskly so that you can improve your cardiovascular health and tone your muscles.

As you walk you should inhale deeply to take in more oxygen.

Walking will also help you to build bone density and protect you from osteoporosis. This is important because when you have strong bones, they will not fracture easily when you fall.

Walking your dog is also a good form of exercise. Both you and your dog will benefit and enjoy better health.

If you cannot exercise in the morning, then do so in the evening.

If you work and cannot find the time to walk, this is what you can do.

Instead of taking the lift or elevator, walk up the stairs. If your office is located on a very high floor, you can get off three or four floors below and walk up the rest of the way.

You can also build up your endurance slowly by climbing more and more stairs each week. This will increase your stamina and muscle strength.

Some people may find it boring to do the same exercise every day. If this is the case, you can do different types of exercise on different days. For example, you can walk on Monday, Wednesday and Friday and cycle or swim on Tuesday, Thursday and Saturday.

B. Strength Training

This can be done two or three times a week. Use light to moderate weights such as dumb bells. If you find dumb bells expensive, you can use mineral water bottles. Fill them up with water and use them as weights. There are 500 ml bottles and 1.5 litre bottles.

You can also use resistance bands, also known as Thera bands, which you can get from sports shops. There are different colours. Pink is the lightest resistance band. As you get stronger, you can graduate to using bands that have greater resistance. You tie the band to a bar or door knob (the door must be closed so that it will not move when you are pulling the band). Then pull the band, to do different exercises to strengthen different muscles in your body.

An exercise you can do to strengthen your shoulder and arm is to tie the band at waist level to the bar or door knob. With your back to the bar and your arm at your side, keep your elbow straight and pull the band out and then up. Do this ten times, slowly, then repeat with the other arm. Keep your body upright and straight when doing the exercise.

Another exercise is to face the bar, to which the band is attached at waist height, and, keeping your elbow straight, pull the band straight back.

Each exercise is repeated ten times and you need to do three sets of ten repetitions each. In the beginning you may start off with one set. Do the exercise slowly and feel your muscles work as you pull the band.

This is to strengthen your muscles and to prevent lean muscle loss. The more muscle there is, the easier it is to control blood sugar levels, and the easier to lose weight.

C. Stretching

Stretching exercises are important for diabetics because they suffer from premature stiffening of the spine and joints. You need to stretch daily to remain flexible. You also need to stretch before you begin your exercises so as not to injure your muscles or ligaments. You can do simple stretching exercises like those you used to do during physical education lessons in school.

You can also attend a yoga class where you learn how to stretch without doing any injury to yourself.

Remember to enjoy the exercise, so that you will feel motivated to keep on doing it. A tip to keep you going is to have an exercise buddy. You will keep each other motivated as you evaluate the results of your exercise plan.

After a couple of months, you will be able to see the results of your exercise regimen. Not only will you be leaner and more flexible but also healthier and more energetic.

In the next chapter, you will learn to implement another lifestyle change. This will be in your food intake.

Changes You Need to Make in Your Diet

Apart from incorporating regular exercise into your daily life, you need to take a hard look at what you are eating, and make the necessary changes, if you want to prevent Diabetes from taking hold in your life.

If you're already a diabetic and still eating the same kind of food, the same way you did before you were diagnosed with Diabetes, then you're headed down a slippery slope to a premature death.

Ouch, but it's a necessary reminder. The Grim Reaper is never far away when you're a diabetic who does not look after your well-being, but continues with your old lifestyle habit of eating whatever you like, resulting in very high sugar levels.

So to keep the Grim Reaper at bay, you need to make changes in your eating habits. You can no longer afford to eat the way you used to before you were diagnosed with Diabetes.

In fact, by changing your eating habits and making healthier choices in your food, you can control your blood sugar levels and make sure that they do not continue to rise. Furthermore, you can also set your target, to achieve a much lower blood sugar level than you currently have.

Let's take a look at the different types of food that many of us consume, without realising the negative impact that they have on our health.

People who partake of a western diet have an increased risk of developing type 2 Diabetes. This is further escalated if they consume more calories than are needed by the body. They are probably eating the wrong types of food, such as eating more refined carbohydrates instead of high fibre food, eating the wrong type of fat and not eating enough vegetables or fruit which are the major source of antioxidants.

A western diet typically includes the following foods:

Red meat
Processed meat
French fries, potatoes
High fat dairy products
Refined grains
Legumes
Sweets / desserts

An Asian diet usually includes the following:

Rice
Noodles
High fat food such as curries
Deep fried food
Vegetables and legumes
Meat and poultry
Fish
Local sweets / desserts
Fruit

Now let's return to what is considered **healthy eating**.

To ensure that we will have optimal health, in spite of our health situation, we must adopt a **prudent diet**. This means we need to eat more of the following:

Vegetables
Fruit
Fish
Poultry
Whole grains

We need to **reduce fat intake**, such as saturated fats and margarine. We also need to **cut down on meat**, especially red meat. Studies have confirmed that a higher intake of meat and animal products leads to an increased risk of diabetes, cancer and heart disease. Meat does not contain any antioxidants or phytochemicals. Instead, they contain saturated fat and harmful compounds, especially when they are grilled, fried or broiled. We should avoid processed meat like bacon, hot dogs, fat-laden meat, especially when they are well-done or charbroiled.

On the other hand, we should increase our intake of Omega 3 fatty acids which are found in fish and flaxseed oil. The fish should be cold water fish such as salmon, mackerel, herring, halibut and anchovies.

Also recommended is an increased intake of mono unsaturated fatty acids or Omega 9 which can be found in olive oil and nuts. **Olive oil** protects against heart disease. It lowers the bad cholesterol also known as LDL and increases the level of HDL or the good cholesterol. It also **improves insulin sensitivity** and contributes to a **better control of blood sugar levels.**

Nuts are rich in fibre and magnesium. It is advisable to eat them raw or lightly roasted. Fresh nuts are preferable to commercial roasted and salted nuts.

Fruit, such as citrus fruits and berries, should be consumed because they contain antioxidants, phytochemicals, Vitamin C and Folic acid, which help to prevent some of the complications leading from Diabetes.

Vegetables such as carrots, dark green leafy vegetables, kale, collards and spinach contain carotene, chlorophyll and flavonoids which protect against free radical damage that could lead to cancer.

Let's replace unhealthy food with **healthy food choices** that will improve our health.

1. **Red meat**: try not to eat more than twice in a month. Eat more fish and poultry instead. (White meat).

2. **High fat dairy products:** Substitute with low fat or non-fat products.

3. **Fried food and fatty snacks:** Eat more vegetables and salads instead.

4. **Hamburgers and hot dogs:** Substitute with vegetarian or soy based products.

5. **Butter, lard and other saturated fats:** Replace with olive oil, coconut oil, or canola oil.

6. **Margarine, and shortening:** Use olive oil and coconut oil instead.

7. **Carbonated drinks and sodas, sweet soft drinks**: Substitute with fresh vegetable and fruit juices, green tea and plain water.

8. **Salt and salty food:** Replace with low salted food and light salt if you must have salt.

9. **Pies, cakes, pastries, cookies, biscuits, ice-creams**: Eat fresh fruit instead. They contain less calories and more nutrients.

Food that is highly recommended for people with Pre-diabetes and Diabetes are those that have a **low glycemic index**.

What is the Glycemic Index?

It is a measure of the speed of the rise in the level of blood sugar, after eating a particular food, and it reveals how quickly a particular food turns into blood sugar.

Foods with a low glycemic index are good for diabetics because they can help with blood sugar control. When you eat food with a lower GI, your blood sugar level will rise slowly, but if you eat food with a high GI, your blood sugar level will rise rapidly.

However, the glycemic index only tells us about the quality of carbohydrates. It doesn't reveal the quantity of carbohydrate in a particular food. The glycemic load (GL) of food is a number that estimates how much the food will raise a person's blood sugar level after eating it. Carbohydrates have adverse effects on blood sugar levels. So knowing both the GI and GL of a particular food will make it easier for a diabetic to choose the type of food he should eat, in order to have a better control of his blood sugar level. The lower the GL, the more suitable it is for a diabetic. He should consider adding that particular food to his diet. The pre-diabetic will be able to normalize his blood sugar if he makes the right selection of food to eat.

In the next chapter, you will get to know the **GI** and **GL** of particular foods.

The Glycemic Index and Glycemic Load of Foods

It is impossible to list all of the different types of food that contain carbohydrate here, so the tables show only foods with high carbohydrate content. Fish, poultry and meat are excluded because they have little carbohydrates. Nuts are also excluded.

Low GI   1-55

Mid GI   56-69

High GI 70 and above

Low GL   1-10

Mid GL   11-19

High GL   20 and above

We'll begin with Breakfast, the most important meal of the day. Included in the tables below are the common foods we usually eat in a **western diet**.

Breakfast

Cereals		GI	GL
All Bran	½ cup	42	9.2
Coco Puffs	1 cup	77	20
Corn Flakes	1 cup	84	21.8
Oatmeal cooked	1 cup	42	10
Raisin bran	1 cup	73	25.5
Rice Krispies	1 cup	82	22

Bread		GI	GL
Bagel	170gm	72	25
Croissant	150gm	67	18
French Baguette	30gm	95	14

Bread		GI	GL
Gluten-free multigrain	1 slice 30gm	79	12
Hamburger bun	150gm	61	15
Multigrain unsweetened	1 slice 30gm	43	4
Pita	1 piece 65gm	57	22
White wheat	1 slice 35gm	69	9.6
White wheat flour	1 slice 30gm	70	10.5

Jam		GI	GL
Jam unsweetened	1 tbsp	55	6
Jam sweetened	1 tbsp	48	8

Cakes		GI	GL
Banana cake	1 slice 80gm	47	21.6
Cupcake with icing	1 cake	73	19

Cakes		GI	GL
Donut, glazed	1 ring 75gm	76	24.3
Flan	1 slice 80gm	65	35.8
Lamingtons	150gm	87	25
Pound cake	1 slice 80gm	54	22.6
Scones	140gm	92	83
Sponge cake	1 slice 60gm	46	14.7

Muffins/pancake		GI	GL
Apple muffin	180gm	44	19
Blueberry muffin	180gm	59	24
Buckwheat pancake	40gm	102	30
Pancake from dry mix	1 large 80gm	67	39

Milk, Soy milk		GI	GL
Low fat milk, chocolate flavour	1 cup 250ml	34	7.8

Milk, Soy milk		GI	GL
Skim milk	1 cup 250ml	32	4
Soy milk	1 cup 250ml	31	3.7
Whole milk	1 cup 250ml	27	3
Nesquik chocolate powder	3 tsp in 250ml milk	55	7.7
Sweetened condensed milk	½ cup 160gm	61	55

Juices		GI	GL
Apple juice unsweetened	1 cup 250ml	40	13.2
Cranberry juice cocktail	240ml	68	23
Orange juice	1 cup 250ml	46	9.7
Pineapple juice, canned, unsweetened	1 cup 250ml	46	12.4
Grapefruit juice, unsweetened	1 cup 250ml	48	7.7

Drinks		GI	GL
Coca cola	375ml	63	25.2
Gatorade	1 cup 250ml	78	11.7
Soft drink	375ml	68	34.7

Now we come to the **main meals**. The food in the tables below are separated into Western and Asian food.

Western		GI	GL
Fettucini, cooked	1 cup 180gm	32	18.2
Macaroni and cheese, cooked	220gm	64	19.2
Pasta	1 cup 180gm	35	15.7
Rice pasta brown, cooked	1 cup 180gm	92	52
Ravioli, meat-filled	1 cup 220gm	39	11.7
Spaghetti gluten-free in tomato sauce	1 small can 220gm	68	18.5

Western		GI	GL
Spaghetti, white, cooked	1 cup 180gm	41	23
Spaghetti, whole-meal cooked	1 cup 180gm	37	17.8
Tortellini, cheese	180gm	50	10.5

Soups		GI	GL
Black bean	220ml	64	6
Lentil canned	220ml	44	6
Split peas, canned	220ml	60	8
Tomato, canned	220ml	38	6

Asian Diet

Most Asians do not partake of a western diet although they do have some food in common such as vegetables and fruits. The tables below indicate the type of food that is usually eaten by Asians.

Breakfast

Bread		GI	GL
White wheat flour	1 slice 30gm	70	10.5
Multigrain unsweetened	1 slice 30gm	69	9.6

Jam		GI	GL
Jam unsweetened	1 tbsp	55	6
Jam sweetened	1 tbsp	48	8

Main Meals		GI	GL
Parboiled rice	1 cup 180gm	47	17
Rice noodles, boiled	1 cup 176gm	40	17.5

Main Meals		GI	GL
Sweet potatoes	1 medium size	61	17
White rice	1 cup 180gm	64	23

The following foods are common in both the Asian and Western diets.

Beans		GI	GL
Baked beans	½ cup	48	10
Black beans	½ cup	45	5.7
Chick peas	½ cup	42	6.3
Kidney beans	½ cup	52	6.7
Lentils	½ cup	28	5.3
Peas	½ cup	48	2
Soy beans	½ cup	14	1.6

Vegetables		GI	GL
Beets, canned, drained	2-3 slices, 60gm	64	3
Carrots, peeled, boiled	½ cup 70gm	49	1.5

Diabetes

Vegetables		GI	GL
Carrots, raw	½ cup 80gm	16	1
Corn, canned, drained	½ cup 80gm	55	8.5
French fries, fine cut	120gm	75	36
Gnocchi, cooked	1 cup 145gm	68	48
Parsnips, boiled	½ cup 75 gm	97	8
Potato, no fat, oven-baked	1 medium 120gm	93	14
Potatoes, instant prepared	½ cup 120gm	83	15
Potatoes, mashed	½ cup 120gm	91	14
Potatoes, new, boiled unpeeled	5 small 175gm	78	20
Potato, with skin, boiled	1 medium 120gm	79	11
Potato, peeled, boiled	1 medium 120gm	87	10
Pumpkin, peeled, boiled	½ cup 85gm	75	4.5
Sweet corn on cob, boiled	80gm	48	8

The following are **low glycemic vegetables**. One cup cooked or raw has a GI of approximately 20 and a GL of approximately 1.4.

Asparagus, Bell peppers, Broccoli, Brussel sprouts, Cabbage, Cauliflower, Cucumber, Celery, Eggplant, Green beans, Kale, Lettuce, Mushrooms, Spinach, Tomatoes, Zucchini.

Fresh Fruit		GI	GL
Apple	1 medium, 150gm	38	6.8
Apricots	3 medium, 100gm	57	4
Banana raw	1 medium 150gm	55	17.6
Cherries	20, 80gm	22	2.2
Grapes, green	1 cup, 100gm	46	6.9
Kiwi, peeled	80gm	52	4
Mango	1 small, 150gm	55	10.4
Orange	1, 130gm	44	4.4
Peach	1, 110gm	42	3
Pear	1, 150gm	38	8
Pineapple	2 slices, 125gm	66	6.6

Fresh Fruit		GI	GL
Plums	3-4 small	39	2.7
Watermelon	11 cup 150gm	72	5.7

Dried Fruit		GI	GL
Apple	30gm	29	6.9
Apricots	5-6 pieces, 30gm	31	4
Dates	5, 40gm	104	27.8
Figs	50gm	61	13.4
Prunes, pitted	6, 40gm	29	7.3
Raisins	¼ cup, 40gm	64	18
Sultanas	¼ cup, 40gm	56	16.8

Canned Fruit		GI	GL
Apricots	½ cup, 125gm	64	8.3
Fruit cocktail	1 cup, 125gm	55	8.3
Peaches	½ cup, 125gm	38	4.5
Pears	½ cup, 125gm	43	5.5

Ice Cream		GI	GL
Vanilla, low fat	100m	38	5.7
Full fat	2 scoops	61	6.1

Sugars		GI	GL
Honey	½ tbsp 10gm	58	4.6
Table sugar	2 tsp	68	7

Biscuits		GI	GL
Breton wheat crackers	6, 25gm	67	9.4
Graham crackers	1, 30gm	74	16
Kavli crackers	4, 20gm	71	9.2
Premium soda crackers	3, 25gm	74	12.5
Ryvita or Wasa	2, 20gm	69	11

Snacks		GI	GL
Corn chips Doritos	50gm	42	13.9
Mars bar	60gm	65	22.6
Pretzels	50gm	83	18.3

Snacks		GI	GL
Real fruit bars, strawberry	20gm	90	15.3
Skittles	62gm	70	38.5
Snickers	59gm	41	14.3

Note: You can find out more information about the glycemic index from this website: http://www.glycemicindex.com/

So by choosing carefully the types of food that you eat, you can lower the level of your blood sugar significantly.

You need to plan your meals by taking into consideration the GI and GL of particular foods so that you can achieve the blood sugar level target which you have set. Pay attention to the serving sizes.

The lower the GL the better it is for those who are diabetic. **A GL of 20 is high, a GL of 11-19 is medium and a GL of 10 or less is low**. Bear in mind that although the GI of a particular food may be high, its GL may be low. So as long as you eat a smaller portion of it, its impact on blood sugar is acceptable.

Try to avoid eating too many carbohydrates. They are not good for diabetics. If you like foods that are high in carbohydrates, then eat a smaller portion. Asians, who eat rice as their staple, can opt for brown rice instead of white rice, which has a high GI. You can also compromise by mixing brown rice with a smaller proportion of white rice when you cook it. However, you would need to adjust the amount of water used in cooking it.

It is highly recommended that you eat more small meals throughout the day than the three main meals. The reason behind this is to keep your metabolism going at a steady rate throughout the day, burning calories, which translates into weight loss.

What are these small meals?

Breakfast is the first meal of the day which you must never skip. It revs up your metabolic rate and gives you the energy to begin your day. Skipping breakfast is a bad idea because it will lead to weight gain in the long run. Your hunger pangs will drive you to eat foods that are sweet, to provide the energy your body needs. Sweet foods are calorie-laden and lack nutrients.

Then you can have a **mid-morning break** followed later by a **light lunch**. By **mid-afternoon**, you are ready for a **snack**. **Dinner** follows later, but no later than at least four hours before your bed time. This is to allow your food to digest before you go to sleep.

I will share with you some examples of what you can include in your daily meals. However, by looking at the tables above, you can create delicious meals for yourself. Just remember to include lots of vegetables as they have very low GI and GL and they contain nutrients which are good for you.

Sample of a Day's Meals

Breakfast

- Fruit: 1 medium-size banana
- Cereal: Oat meal (sweetened with ½ tbsp. honey)
- 2 slices unsweetened multi-grained bread with 1 tbsp. jam
- 1 cup coffee/tea, preferably unsweetened

Mid-morning break

- 1 medium-size apple
- 2 pieces Ryvita biscuit
- 1 cup tea/coffee, unsweetened (optional or substitute with fruit juice)

Lunch

- 1 medium-size orange
- Mixed vegetable salad
- 2 chicken sandwiches with tomatoes and lettuce
- 1 cup tea/coffee (this can be substituted with warm water)

Afternoon break

- 1 cup hot chocolate 250ml (unsweetened)
- 1 muffin

Dinner

- 1 medium-size pear
- Tomato soup
- 1 grilled chicken chop with carrot & broccoli
- 1 medium-size oven-baked potato (no fat)
- 1 scoop ice cream (optional)
- 1 cup tea/coffee (unsweetened)

Note: **Fruit should be taken before meals, on an empty stomach.**

Bonus Tips to Lower Your Blood Sugar Levels and Manage Your Diabetes

1. When cooking, do not use butter. Use olive oil instead. It's healthier and protects your heart.

2. Avoid mayonnaise or Thousand Island Dressing in your salad. Opt for balsamic vinegar.

3. If you like Asian meals, cut down on the amount of rice or noodles. Have bigger portions of vegetables, whether stir-fried or boiled. Opt to steam your fish and poultry rather than deep-fry.

4. Plan your meals 3 days in advance and pin your planner on your refrigerator door so that you can see at a glance, what you're going to eat for a particular day.

5. Keep a food diary so that you have a record of what you eat each day. This is useful because if your blood sugar reading suddenly spikes, you can refer to what you ate the previous day so that you will know which food most likely caused that spike. You can then be careful and limit the intake of that particular food or omit it from your diet altogether.

A. Juices that reduced my blood sugar levels

I use **bitter gourd** (the small, very bitter variety) as the main ingredient. Bitter gourd reduces blood sugar levels by increasing glucose utilisation in the liver.

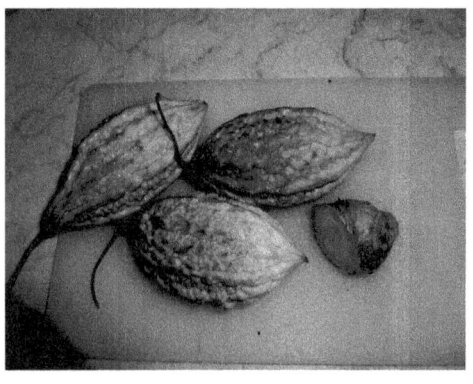

3 small bitter gourds
1 small knob of ginger
2 stalks celery
1 green apple
1 cup fresh pineapple

Juice the above and drink immediately before the juice oxidises.

Celery, bitter gourd and green apple are the main items and I rotate the pineapple and ginger with carrot and lemon.

Sometimes I use cucumber, ginger, bitter gourd, green apple and guava.

How often do I juice?

Every morning initially, but now it's alternate days, since my blood sugar levels are on target.

B. Natural teas that reduce blood sugar and high blood pressure.

There are herbs that bring down blood sugar levels and high blood pressure. I use **mulberry leaves** and the leaves known as **Cat's Whiskers** or the very bitter **Snake grass**. These leaves are taken separately. For example, I may drink Mulberry tea for a week, then Cat's Whiskers tea the following week.

The leaves are boiled for about 20 minutes and left to cool. Then I drink it throughout the day. If I don't have the time to boil it, I just infuse the dried leaves with hot water. You can air-dry the leaves in a cool spot in your home.

Drinking these teas regularly brings down the sugar levels. I know, because I monitor my blood sugar level every few days, using a glucometer to check.

C. A vegetable known as Okra or Ladies' Fingers can also help to reduce blood sugar levels.

This is a folk remedy recommended by the elders. Take 3 to 4 pieces of Okra and make a few cuts on the vegetable. Then leave to soak overnight in a cup of water. When you wake up the next morning, on an empty stomach, drink the water and discard the vegetable. Take your sugar level reading before trying out this remedy. After a few weeks, check your blood sugar level again.

See if it has dropped.

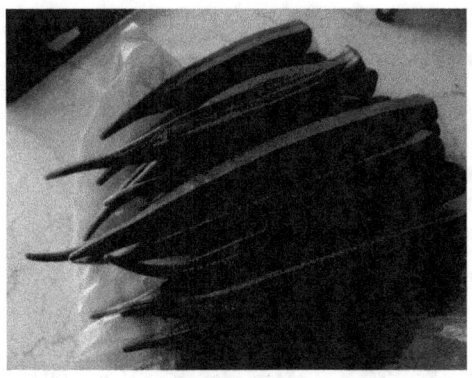

Okra

D. Other helpful herbs and spices

a. Gymnema:

This herb decreases the absorption of sugar from the intestine. It suppresses sweet cravings, thus encouraging weight loss. It also increases cell growth in the pancreas, thus raising the amount of insulin produced.

b. Tumeric:

This spice contains curcumin, which reduces fasting blood sugar and helps to regulate it. The American Diabetic Association's journal, *Diabetes Care*, published a study which found that turmeric extract successfully prevented pre-diabetics from developing Diabetes. It also improves cell function in the pancreas, thereby increasing insulin production and sensitivity.

c. Cinnamon:

A study published in the Diabetes Care Journal found that cinnamon improves blood glucose and cholesterol levels in people with type 2 diabetes. Another study revealed that an intake of 1 gm of cinnamon a day increases insulin sensitivity and helps in the management of Diabetes.

If you're already a diabetic, you would want to keep your fasting blood sugar level below 7.0mmol/L. This is my target as I was already a confirmed diabetic when I saw the doctor. Sometimes, my sugar levels drop below 6 to 5.6 or 5.8, depending on what I ate the previous day. However, if I ate something very sweet, e.g. grapes in the evening, then my blood sugar level would go beyond 7 but never up to 9.0. So I'm cautious and avoid eating grapes. I now maintain my sugar level at a steady range of between 5.8 to 6.2 although it might go up to 6.6 if I had something sweet the night before.

How Can You Check Your Blood Sugar Level?

You can purchase a glucometer from a pharmacy. Tell the pharmacist that you want to monitor your blood sugar levels. He will tell you what you need to purchase. The kit includes lancets and a lancing device to which you attach the lancet so that you can prick your finger to get a tiny drop of blood.

You will also need alcohol swabs to clean your finger before you prick it and a box of glucose test strips.

Here's a picture of what you need before you do your test.

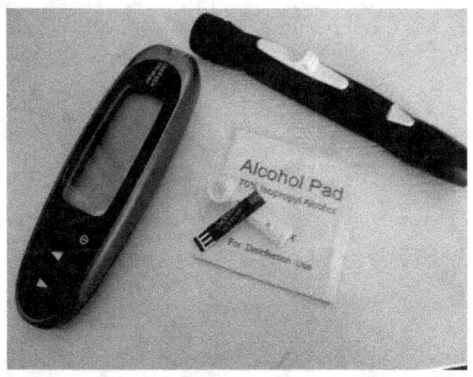

First, you insert the test strip into the meter. The code will flash on the screen of the meter. You need to make sure the code is similar to the code on the box of your test strips. The booklet that comes with your meter will show you how to make sure the codes match.

Insert the lancet into the lancing device. Then swab your finger with the alcohol pad. When it is dry, lance your finger tip. A small drop of blood will appear. Hold the tip of the test strip to the blood so that it runs into the strip. The meter will then give you a reading. That will be your blood sugar level.

Record your blood sugar level in the notebook that comes with your meter. Note the date, time of test and the reading. Discard the used strip and lancet. Each time you do a test, you must record the results so that you can track your blood sugar levels.

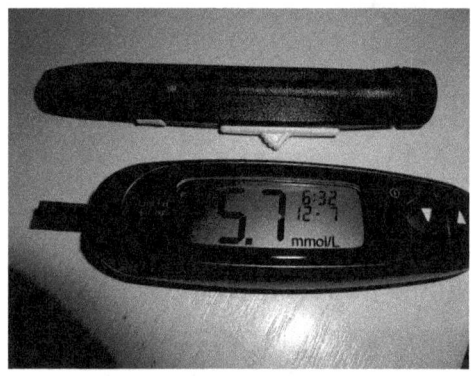

The above shows my fasting blood sugar level reading on the morning of 7th July, 2016, taken at 06:32. It is 5.7mmol/L.

So far we've seen the importance of keeping blood sugar levels within a safe limit. What happens if your blood sugar levels go too low? Yes, this can happen too.

Any blood sugar level reading below 72md/dL or 4.0mmol/L indicates hypoglycaemia.

Hypoglycemia can come on suddenly. It is usually triggered by a delay in having a meal or missing a meal, drinking alcohol (while under medication or insulin therapy) or exercising too long or too strenuously. If left untreated, it can result in coma, brain damage and death.

What are the symptoms of hypoglycemia?

A person who is hypoglycemic feels weak and tired. Their heart beats rapidly and they begin to tremble. They perspire and their sweat is cold. They also feel dizzy, confused, nauseous and they might have a headache too.

To prevent them from losing consciousness, their sugar levels need to be raised immediately. So you have to give them some sweets or candy. If sweet fruit juice is available, give them half a cup to restore their sugar levels to normal. Then, as soon as possible, they need to have a snack or a meal.

This actually happened to my friend while we were playing golf. He's diabetic. We knew that, but he'd never had any problem before.

There were four of us in a flight and we were on the second nine, having completed the first, in very hot weather. My friend suddenly felt faint and he was perspiring a great deal, more than usual. We could see that he was unwell. He asked if we had any sweets on us. Fortunately, one of us did. So we gave him the sweets and he felt better after that. He refused to return to the clubhouse and insisted on completing the round as we had only another two holes to go. Once we completed the game, and adjourned to the clubhouse, we had a light meal and he recovered completely. It had been the hot weather, and he had skipped his breakfast earlier that morning. That was a very foolish thing to do.

It is advisable for a diabetic to carry a packet of sweets, especially when exercising. One can never know what might happen.

So far we have talked about two lifestyle changes that you must make in order to manage and control your blood sugar levels, i.e. incorporating an exercise regimen in your daily life and making changes in your food choices.

In the next chapter, you will learn more about other lifestyle changes which you need to adopt, so that you will be healthy and enjoy a better quality of life.

Other Important Life Style Changes

1. Change your bad habits

Smoking, drinking, and regular late nights are bad habits which you need to break. They directly impact your sugar levels.

If you already have Diabetes and still continue to smoke, your blood sugar levels will be much higher, making it more difficult for you to control. You will be at greater risk of developing complications such as blindness, nerve damage, kidney failure and heart problems. In fact, you have a very great risk of having a heart attack!

So this is one habit you need to kick!

Drinking can lead to becoming overweight and eventually obesity. I'm sure you are familiar with scenes where people quaff down bottles of beer or hard liquor, accompanied by munching on crisps, peanuts and other junk food. Little do they realize that they could develop Diabetes if they keep on doing this, over a period of time. If a diabetic is suffering from nerve pain, consuming alcohol will make it worse.

Drinking, smoking, and eating nutrient empty food, plus regular late nights will take a toll on your health. Sleep deprivation, or insufficient sleep, will affect your body's hormone levels and compromise its ability to regulate and metabolize glucose.

When your blood sugar level is really high, your kidneys try to excrete it through urine. This means that your sleep will be disturbed as you will be going to the bathroom a few times in the night to urinate.

Remember, poor quality sleep and lack of sleep can lead to obesity and diabetes.

If you're not a diabetic, sleep deprivation could lead to Prediabetes. You should try to get at least 6 hours' sleep if you can't manage to get 8 hours at a stretch.

2. Don't let stress and anxiety take the joy out of your life.

Maintain a balance in your life. You may have problems at work, or on the home front but you need to keep them in perspective. Make time for your family. What was not completed in the office, can be continued the next day. The time you spend with your family will pay dividends. It will enhance family bonding and lead to a happy family.

Relax after a day's work. Destress by going for a walk. Listen to soothing music. When you are relaxed, it will enable you to enjoy better sleep.

3. Management of Diabetes

a. Make it a habit to check your blood sugar levels regularly and keep a food diary.

b. See your doctor every four months for regular monitoring of your Diabetes. He will send you for a blood test to check on your kidney function, to see if your blood sugar levels are under control and also to check if there is any albumin in your urine. This is important as it may indicate kidney disease. He may also order an HbA1c test which gives the average blood sugar levels over a period of three months. This will indicate whether your blood sugar levels are under control or not.

c. He may prescribe medication if your sugar levels are not well-controlled. If so, you need to take your medication regularly so that the disease will not progress to a stage where complications set in.

d. Have regular foot examination, preferably quarterly checks. You need to check for ulcers and any abnormalities in the toe nails. Exercise care to avoid any injury to your feet. Make sure your footwear is comfortable. Shop for shoes in the afternoon as that's when your feet are at their biggest! Feet tend to swell in the afternoon, so when you buy your shoes at that time, you will be sure of a good fit. If you purchase in the morning, you will find that your feet are no longer comfortable in your new shoes come afternoon.

e. Go for sensory tests to rule out nerve damage.

    f.   You also need an annual eye examination to check on your optic nerve and retina. As we age, macular degeneration takes place. Be mindful that Diabetes can lead to blindness so an eye examination by the eye specialist is very important.

    g.   Above all, you should maintain an ideal weight and stick to your exercise program.

Management and medication are important because you don't want your Diabetes to get worse than it already is. You want to arrest it and maintain at that level or try to lower your blood sugar levels.

A careful monitoring of your blood sugar levels, eating habits and diet management plus a regular exercise regimen will enable you to lead a comfortable and healthy life and you can look forward to a longer life span. Think what that means!!

You can see your grandchildren grow up and you get to enjoy them. If you are retired, you can do all the things you never got to do while you were working full time. So with that in mind, I'm sure you don't need further prodding to lead a healthy lifestyle and to keep Diabetes at bay or under good control.

Don't Forget My Gift for You

Thank you again for reading my book. As a token of appreciation, I would like to give you a list of the Glycemic Index of food which you can download and print out. This will help you to make healthy choices when grocery shopping for your meals.

To get your gift, go to:

http://www.peggychan.online/gi-food-list-signup/

Acknowledgements

I would like to take the opportunity to thank my family and friends for their support and encouragement in my passion for writing.

Thanks also go to those worked behind the scenes, who helped to make this book a reality, the cover designers, the editor and formatter. I'm grateful to the community in the Self-Publishing School for their encouragement and help in getting this book out into the world!

Last but not least I would like to thank my readers, who read my books. Without them and their support there would be no books, so to speak!

About the Author

Peggy is a happy grandmother of four, two of whom are in college, and two of whom are pre-schoolers. She enjoys an early morning round of golf, travelling and creative writing. Reading is what she likes to do best when not bogged down with the mundane routines of life.

She has published English Grammar books and also a series of "Yes I Can Read" stories retold in simple language for children.

You can find her other books, both fiction and non-fiction, including children's books, in the Kindle store on amazon.com.

She shares the places she has visited and her thoughts in her blogs at blogger.com

You are welcome to check them out at:

https://swingingby.blogspot.my/
https://bubblyluv.blogspot.my/

More from Peggy

If you enjoyed reading this book, please sign up to my reader list to get more information and promotions on my books. Hear about my latest books before anyone else.

Join my Readers List at:
http://www.peggychan.online

And you will get this book, absolutely free – available for immediate download!

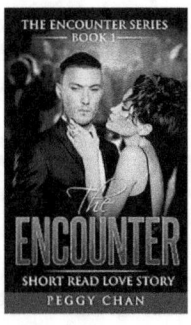

Thank You for Downloading and Reading This Book!

I appreciate your feedback and would love to hear what you have to say.

Your input is needed and would be most helpful to make my next book better.

Please leave me a helpful review on Amazon by going to:

https://www.amazon.com/dp/B01LXBUBNO

Thank you very much!